How to Love Your Hair & Hair Extensions

By Mandy Allen

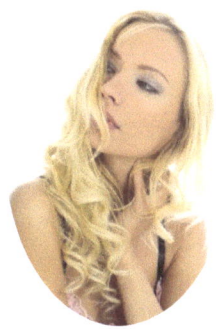

The must have manual on caring for your hair and hair extensions. Everything you need to know about hair extensions.

Long, thick and luscious hair is not just a dream ... it is ABSOLUTELY achievable!

You can also save money, with my hair care tips. It all comes down to understanding your hair, knowing when it needs a little extra TLC. Learn how to look after your own hair and hair extensions to ensure they both last longer, look and feel fabulous! Learn how to shop for the best quality hair extensions, understand the hair extension industry lingo - Grading, Quality, and Hair Types. Shop for hair extension methods that will fit your lifestyle.

Contents

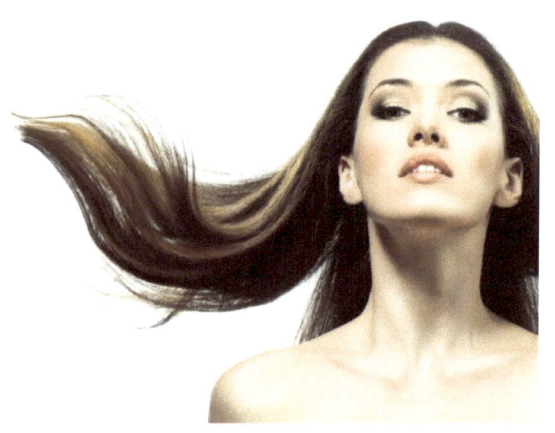

BEHIND THE SCENES

The faces behind Hollywood Glamour hair extension business ... Mandy Allen and Gavin Roake, directors of Hollywood Glamour.

About me ... Mandy, 36 years young, and I have spent all of those years surrounded by wigs, hair pieces and hair extensions, the beauty industry in general, with my mother also being a qualified beautician . Yes we are a family owned business .

Where we began .... about 40 or 50 years ago, with my father who arrived in New Zealand, got his business started the good old fashioned way. Approaching all those he saw on the street he felt could do with a hairpiece. My father not blessed with diplomacy in his youth... earned himself a few bleeding noses, and black eyes, with his opening line "I can help you get your hair back" to balding young men on the street. His technique whilst not diplomatic, did build up his business.

Over the years the business expanded to include hair extensions. As a child I remember spending the school holidays in my parents shop, which to, many young children this may have seemed exciting, trying on funky wigs, and hair extensions. We found it rather boring after years of spending spare moments at my parents shop ... and when I left home I swore I would NEVER enter the family business.

Years ago hair extensions were manufactured with Synthetic hair, that would matt and look tragic after a few wears. They were all attached to a banana clip, or some sort of hair tie, which was completely limiting on style. About 8 years ago, my mother trying to reel me into the family business decided the best way forward would be just to courier me some clip in hair extensions. Well that was it ... the turning point! Hair Extensions had moved forward leaps and bounds, now high quality human hair, I could curl , straighten them, and style my hair extensions however I like.

What can I say - I'm in love with hair extensions - sign me up for the family business! And would you believe this is exactly what happened!

After working alongside my mother for a few years, and having extended myself fully into the hair extension industry, she offered me the entire company, this time I gladly accepted. I had found my passion, my dream.

We are now based in Auckland, New Zealand and solely focus on manufacturing the highest quality premium human hair extensions.

I personally wear our hair extensions, tape in hair extensions being my absolute favourite method of permanent extensions I have ever tried - unbelievably comfortable, you completely forget you are wearing hair extensions.

On a daily basis we get calls from clients trying to better understand hair extensions, and how to purchase exactly what they are wanting in hair extensions - from length to volume, to styling and ensuring that the hair extension method they have chosen will fit their lifestyle.

It is for this reason I have decided to write a book to help those wanting hair extensions to understand all the industry lingo to ensure when you buy, you are getting exactly what you are after.

Along the way I will not only educate you on Hair types and grading, caring for your hair extensions and keeping a healthy hair balance, but give you my own personal tips to keeping your hair and hair extensions looking fabulous!

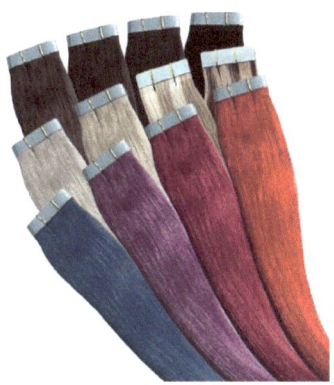

UNDERSTANDING THE HAIR

Understanding you hair is half the battle, knowing when it needs a little extra protein or moisture can make all the difference to your hair's manageability, look and feel. And there are simple tests you can do at home to help you know just what sort of TLC your hair needs.

Healthy Hair Balance

Your hair is not living, which means that it cannot repair itself, however that doesn't mean that you can't.

Healthy hair balance is crucial to your hairs health, look and manageability. Understanding hair's requirements is half the battle.

Healthy hair requires 4 balances

1. Protein
2. Moisture
3. Natural Oils
4. pH Balance

Healthy hair when wet will stretch slightly and return to its normal length with no breakage.

Every week I see clients that come to me with hair care problems, generally they have spent excessive amounts of money on hair care products that is making absolutely no difference purely because they do not understand what the cause of their hair care issues are, and what their hair is lacking.

It is extremely important you understand your hair to be able to treat and nourish it.

Remember the old saying 'too much of a good thing can be bad' - it is so true when it comes to your hair!

When dealing with hair extensions it is even more important to understand your hair's needs as environment, heat, chemicals, all affects our hair's natural balance, and your hair extensions have no natural oils going through your hair daily to help combat these factors, so keeping a healthy hair balance will ensure the longevity of your human hair extensions and will help you grow your own hair too.

Your hair's natural balance will be affected by the environment you expose your hair too (chemicals, heat, pollutants), products you apply and your diet - the old saying you are what you eat is so true! But that's for another book.

Protein

Did you know that your hair is made from a Protein called Keratin?

This gives our hair it's strength and structure, and it is important that we maintain healthy protein levels in our hair to help rebuild and reinforce the hair strands.

Hair's optimum protein level is between 83-87%. If your hair is lacking in protein, it will lack strength and break easily. If you are wanting to retain and grow your hair's length then you need to retain your hair's protein levels.

TIP ... WET HAIR TEST (PROTEIN)

If your hair is very stretchy when it is wet, or it is breaking, then your hair is lacking Protein. Weak, spongy or limp hair when wet are also signals that your hair is in desperate need of protein.

Moisture

Your hair is about 3% moisture. Although moisture only makes up 3% of our hair it is still extremely important. Hair that is lacking in moisture often appears dry, brittle, hard and ridged, and lacks shine.

Did you know that moisture is responsible for our hair's elasticity?

TIP ... WET HAIR TEST (MOISTURE)

When your hair is wet if there is very little or no stretching and the hair breaks, your hair is lacking in moisture. If your hair feels rough, hard, brittle this is also a sign of lack of moisture.

How To Add Moisture or Protein Into Your Hair

There are many ways of getting extra moisture or protein into your hair. When you buy hair product from your local salon, some products are specifically designed for adding moisture and others for adding protein.

1 STEAM - if you have a hair steamer, sit under it for 15-30 minutes. Steam lifts your hair cuticle and infuses the hair shaft with moisture. L'Oreal Steampod machine is also a fantastic way to get steam into your hair and open up the hair shaft.

2 PRODUCT - Use a quality salon shampoo and conditioner. Look for a quality hair mask. Hair masks are more intense than conditioners and will add more moisture or protein to your hair.

TIP … When washing your hair, shampoo it twice. This will remove any build up in your hair, thus improving your hair's ability to accept moisture.

3 FOR AN INTENSIVE TREATMENT - apply a hair mask to your damp hair, and either put a shower cap over your hair, or wrap your hair with a damp hot towel and leave on for 10-15 minutes. You will instantly feel the difference.

Natural Oils

Did you know hair is very porous and has trouble keeping moisture in?

This is why natural oils are so important. Oils do not actually moisturize the hair, they are used to seal the hair to ensure the moisture is retained within the hair.

Oils are large molecules that are too large to be absorbed into the hair shaft, therefore they coat the outside of the hair shaft locking moisture in. It is important only to use a light coating of oil.

If you use oils without moisturizing your hair, or if you hair is lacking in moisture, the oil will seal the moisture out of your hair and lead to eventual dryness.

Remember oil will not penetrate your hair shaft, it will simply coat the hair, locking moisture in. Oils give your hair shine, and the illusion of moisture, it does not actually moisturize the hair.

TIP ... Limit the use of Shine products with lots of silicone, as over time the silicone will build up in your hair and leave it looking dull and lifeless.

pH Balance

Your hair's ideal pH balance is between 4.5 -5.5. If your hair has been stripped of its normal pH balance it will also have been stripped of its natural oils. This will leave your hair feeling dry and damaged, and it can appear frizzy.

When looking for a good shampoo look for the pH level on the bottle. If you can't find it, ask the sales assistant, or contact the manufacturer. An ideal pH level for your shampoo is between 4.5 - 6.5.

Summary

As I mentioned before too much of a good thing can be bad. In the case of your hair without the 4 natural balances, an excess or lack or any of these balance can cause your hair to present with the same issues - dryness, breakage, lack of lustre and shine, so understanding your hair's needs is important.

Next time your hair feels like it needs something a little extra do the 'Wet Hair Test' to help you determine what it is your hair really needs. Take the guess work out of it - it could save you a lot of money!

TIP ... If you are still unsure what it is your hair is lacking, try moisture first, and consult a hair professional.

CARING FOR YOUR HAIR

First ... My Absolute Favourite Hair Treat

Having been in the hair industry for years, and tried too many products to count, in recent years I have come to LOVE Virgin Coconut Oil, an <u>affordable</u> hair treat.

Sometimes, those of us in the hair industry can be the worst, we will push our hair to its ultimate limits, radically changing our hair colour far too often, trying to keep up with hair trends. I have found coconut oil to be my hair saviour!

It must be Virgin Coconut oil that you use ... it makes a fantastic deep conditioning hair mask, that repairs your hair from within!

It nourishes your hair and hair extensions leaving them so soft, shiny and healthy.

Most hair care products can only coat the hair surface, and this is where coconut oil differs and is amazing.

Unlike most other oils, with coconut oils chemical molecular structure, it will actually penetrate deep into the cortex (inside) of your hair. It will actually improve your hair and hair extensions strength and flexibility, adding both protein and moisture directly into your hair shaft. If your hair is dry, breaking, damaged, shedding, then I personally recommend Virgin Coconut oil.

Coconut oil will actually improve the health of your hair!

I now use coconut oil twice a week before washing my hair. It has literally saved my long locks from the chemical torture I subject my hair too.

Trust me this is one product your hair will LOVE!

1. It contains Vitamin E which will help rebuild the protein in your hair
2. Strengthens your hair from the inner cortex
3. Gives your hair moisture and shine, leaving it beautifully soft
4. Great for scalp complaints such as dandruff
5. You will immediately see and feel the results!

How to Use Coconut Oil

Work the coconut oil through your hair (dry hair) right to the ends, and leave it on overnight. For longer hair tie it back or plait it. Wash and condition your hair as per normal the next day. If you don't want to leave it on overnight leave it on for a minimum of 30 minutes.

In cold temperatures, coconut oil will go white and solid, so put the jar of coconut oil in a bowl of boiling water or microwave it for approx 20-30 seconds to melt it (time will vary depending on your microwave), or alternatively if you rub some around in your hands it will melt in seconds.

 In warmer temperatures it will be a clear liquid.

* BEAUTY TIP - Did you know you can also use your Virgin Coconut oil to remove your make-up, including waterproof mascara. Your skin will look and feel fabulous!

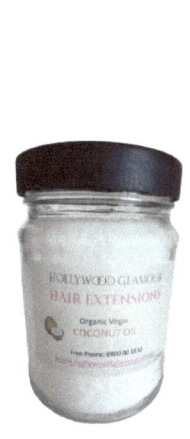

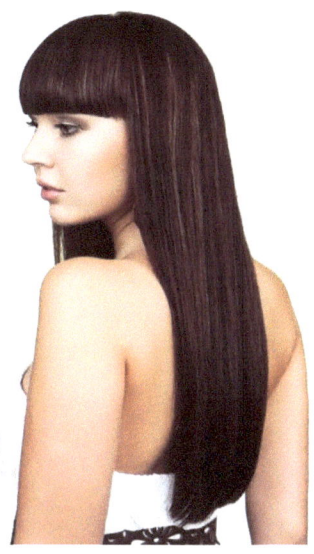

CARING FOR HAIR EXTENSIONS
(and your own hair)

Washing

Only use salon purchased products recommended by your stylist, on your hair extensions. Remember to look for a shampoo with a pH level between 4.5 -6.5.

It is important that you do not use products with high silicone content as this may affect the attachments on permanent hair extensions. It will also affect your hair's ability to absorb moisture, as silicone will coat the hair shaft, locking the moisture out.

Do not use products that contain sulphur, such as dandruff shampoo on hair extensions

For clip in hair extensions wash them in the hand basin. For permanent hair extensions tilt your head back and cleanse from the top of the head downwards. Gently massage shampoo into the scalp and hair being sure not to pull on the hair extensions. Rinse thoroughly and repeat if desired. Do not rub or scrub the hair otherwise matting can occur.

Apply conditioner to the length of your hair, avoiding the root area, apply only to the mid-lengths and ends, comb through with your fingers until hair feels tangle free. Rinse thoroughly. Always leave your conditioner on for the recommended time.

TIP .. When conditioning your permanent hair extensions section your hair into two parts, each side of your face, so you can work the conditioner through your hair and hair extensions using your fingers to comb the conditioner through. If you are not working your conditioner through you are only conditioning the top strands of your hair.

We recommend using a conditioning treatment on the mid-lengths to ends of your hair extensions once a week.

Do not brush the hair while it is wet, always use a wide tooth comb or your fingers.

*BEAUTY TIP - If you run out of shaving cream in the shower, use your hair conditioner, it will lubricate your skin, and leave soft and smooth.

Drying

Do not dry with a scrubbing motion, but instead wrap your hair with a towel to remove moisture. If you have permanent hair extensions, always dry the base area (scalp area where your hair extensions are attached) thoroughly. This is to ensure you don't have any slipping of your hair extensions.
When blow drying your hair and hair extensions use low to medium heat, aim the heat down the hair shaft starting at the root area moving towards the ends, gently moving the hair with your fingers until at least 50% of your hair is dry, then you can introduce brushes to style your hair.

Brushing

Why you really should invest in a Loop hair extension brush ...

If you have hair extensions or even just fine hair that tends to break easily. You really should go and invest in a Loop Brush, you will often find you can get them cheaper than a normal hair brush!

Loop brushes are specifically designed for hair extension wearers, and are fantastic for your own hair also. They are designed to prevent breakage or damage to your hair extensions when brushing your hair.

The loop bristles are much gentler on your hair, keeping your hair extensions tangle free, beautiful and they will last longer!

TIP... Always brush your hair before washing (when dry) to remove any tangles. The reason for doing this is your hair is more elastic and stretchy when wet, and can break easily. By removing any knots and tangles while your hair is dry, reduces breakage, and ensures you can gently and easily work your shampoo and conditioner through your hair.

Sleeping

If you have naturally long hair or permanent hair extensions, you should always loosely plait your hair at night, to prevent your hair from knotting, and to prevent hair breakage. Make sure your hair is completely dry before you go to sleep.

TIP... Always brush your hair before bed, removing any tangles. If you toss and turn a lot in your sleep, or regularly awake with knotty hair invest in silk or satin pillowslip to prevent your hair matting.

Never sleep in clip in extensions, always remove and brush before bed.

Sports

Always tie your hair up before swimming or engaging in sports.

Chlorine or sea water will affect the your natural hair and your hair extensions so it is extremely important to shampoo and condition as directed immediately after such activities to remove any sweat build up in your hair and scalp, and to remove chlorine or salt from your hair.

Products containing Sulphurous substances (e. g thermal baths) can affect attachments of some forms of permanent hair extensions and therefore they should be avoided.

Sports and activities that result in your hair being subjected to a constant, damp environment. For example, regular aerobics, gymnastics, steam baths or saunas may lessen the longevity of the hair extensions, as these constant dampness will weaken the attachments.

TIP ... Wet your hair thoroughly before swimming, as when your hair is wet, the hair shaft expands, hence your hair will absorb less chlorine or salt.

Finishing Products

Avoid using products containing any alcohol, as alcohol can dry out your hair and hair extensions. If you have permanent hair extensions, when using waxes, gels, serums or oils avoid contact with the attachments. Only use these products on the mid lengths to ends of your hair extensions.

Colouring of Hair Extensions

Should only be done by qualified hair dresser who is trained in dealing with human hair extensions. A test strand MUST always be completed first, this is extremely important, as hair extensions are chemically processed hair, the processing time may differ to your own hair, which is why doing a test strand is important to ensure the colour and reflect is correct.

It is usually recommend only colouring your human hair extensions up to 2 shades darker. Keep the colour away from any attachments in permanent extensions.
DO NOT bleach your hair extensions.

PERSONAL NOTE - I would always recommend getting any colouring done by a hairdresser, even your own natural hair. Over the years I have seen many home colouring disasters, and trust me each time it would have worked out a whole lot cheaper for a hairdresser to have coloured their hair originally, than to fix it after a home colouring job!

TIP... If you are working on a budget, discuss this with your hairdresser about what colour choices would allow you to go longer between visits. For example doing a half head of highlights (on top and sides) may make grey hairs less noticeable as your hair grows than if you had a block colour. Choosing shades that are within 1-2 shades of your natural colour near the roots, will make re-growth less obvious.

Heat - Curling, Straightening

Wow, heated styling tools, what a revolution! With this amazing technology though comes the downside of heat damage to your hair, and hair extensions. Human hair extensions are not root-based and therefore do not receive the same nutrients and oils as your natural hair, so you need to be even more aware of heat damage.

Always, always use a heat protector - if you are not kind to your hair in this regard, your hair will pay you back with dryness, damage, knotty and split ends - so make the investment, and get a good quality heat protector!

Be aware, the more you use heat on your hair, the shorter the life-span of the hair extensions. If you do use heat on your hair extensions always use a low setting and apply a Thermal Heat Protector and Shine Serum on them afterwards.

PERSONAL NOTE - I personally have been introduced to and fallen in love with L'Oreal Steampod machine. This revolutionary machine uses steam to straighten and style your hair, with the added bonus of repairing your hair.

When used in conjunction with their Pro-Keratin Cream, the steam activates the ingredients in the cream and repairs your hair, smoothing the hair shaft and sealing the ends.

It leaves both my hair and the hair extensions remarkably soft and shiny.

Maintenance for Permanent Hair Extensions

While you may think that you are saving your wallet a little by stretching out those maintenance appointments with permanent hair extensions, chances are you could be damaging your hair.

Maintenance on permanent hair extensions differs with different types of hair extensions so check with your stylist. Maintenance is to move your hair extensions back closer to your scalp and to keep your extensions looking fresh and to prevent any damage. It also stops any matting near the scalp.

We each lose approx 50-150 hair's a day. If you stretch your maintenance visits past the recommended time, you will have more stress on your natural hair, as some of the hair's in the attachments will no longer be attached to your scalp. Therefore extra pressure is being placed on the remaining hair's in the attachments.

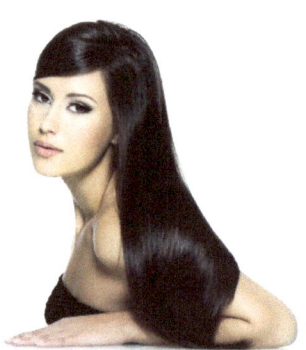

WHY BUY HAIR EXTENSIONS?

Hair Extensions were previously a celebrities best kept hair secrets, now Hollywood stars openly discuss that their fabulous long locks are often hair extensions.

You may feel like you need a hair make over if ...

1. your hair looking a 'little average' (thin or damaged),
2. just simply won't grow
3. you want to add some fun highlights (without adding chemicals)
4. you want stunning length
5. you just love to be able to change and mix up your hairstyles

If you're in need of a hair make over, then hair extensions are probably your answer! Watch out your new look will be very addictive!

The true secret to fabulous hair extensions, is buying quality human hair extensions, that will stay looking great, and last.

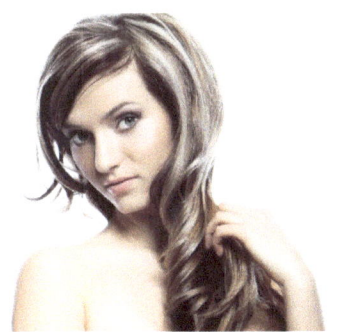

SHOPPING FOR HAIR EXTENSIONS

Shopping for hair extensions can be daunting and confusing, understanding the lingo - Grades, hair types, hair weight. Every week at Hollywood Glamour we get phone calls and emails from people trying to better understand what they are purchasing so, here is the low down - what you need to know to make and educated decision, so that you purchase extensions that are right for you.

Understanding each of these elements is very important, as it effects the quality and longevity of the extensions, thickness, and how the ends of the hair extensions are - thin and spindly, or naturally thick.

Always Buy from a Reputable Supplier

Inferior hair extension suppliers, offering cheap hair extensions will be your worst nightmare!

You don't want to waste your valuable time and money on hair extensions that are going to look tragic after 2-3 washes.

How can that happen you ask?

Some manufacturers will actually mix synthetics, animal hair and fibre's in with their hair extensions, and some just use extremely cheap poor quality hair.

Poor quality hair is normally put through an acid bath, to strip the hair cuticle. The acid bath makes the hair appear thinner, finer, more like the higher quality hair types.

These manufacturers will then coat the hair with silicone. The silicone will make the hair appear soft and shiny, but after a couple of washes the silicone washes off and you are left with the poor quality hair you purchased. Which can be harsh, brittle, dry, breaking, shedding and quite possibly a matted (knotty) mess. What a waste!

Things You Can Do … to ensure you get the best possible hair extensions for your money.

Investigate … the hair extension supplier , they should always be able to tell you about the

1. Hair Quality - Remy, Non Remy
2. Where the hair is sourced from (European, Indian, Asian, etc)
3. What Grade the extensions are (how full they are to the ends)
4. Is the hair sourced ethically?
5. <u>Actual</u> Hair Weight

Check social media sites (not for how many friends or like's they have, but read client testimonials and recommendations on the Hair Extension company). Check home timely the company replies to customer enquiry on social media.

If buying online, check that the company is contactable, address, phone numbers

Check their refund, and exchange policies

Don't be scared to question the company you are planning on purchasing from about where they source the hair from, hair quality and types, etc. Chances are if they can't answer your questions satisfactorily, they do not have enough industry experience to source quality hair, and manufacture quality extensions for you.

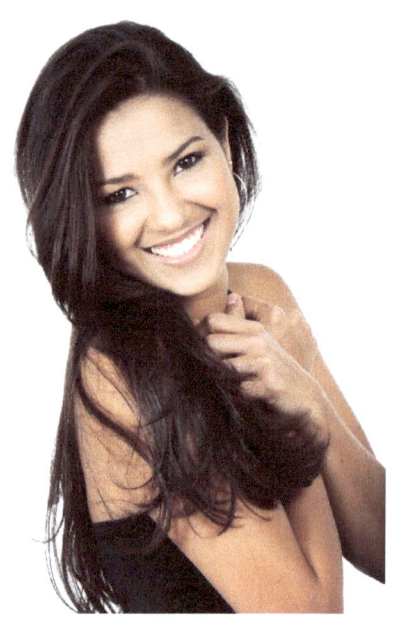

UNDERSTANDING HAIR QUALITY

Never buy hair extensions that are Non Remy! It's that simple!
Well not if you want them last past a couple of washes.

Synthetic Hair

Synthetic hair has a much shorter time span than human hair
(normally 1-2 months). It cannot be re-coloured. Some
synthetics whilst heat friendly most synthetics will melt with the
intensity of heat your straightening/styling tools have.

Human Hair

Human hair with proper care should last up to 1 year or even
longer. Human hair also offers more flexibility when it comes to
styling. It can be curled, straightened (use heat protector), re-
styled, re-coloured and permed. There are two main types of
human hair, which refers to the way in which the hair was
collected, Remy hair and Non Remy hair.

Remy Hair

Remy hair refers to human hair which has been harvested from
root to end, with all of the cuticles going in the same direction.
It is different from Virgin hair as it may be coloured or permed,
but has NOT had the cuticle removed. It is generally soft and
silky, and is used in making higher quality wigs, human hair
extensions, and hair systems.

Remy hair extensions require a careful selection process that has strict controls, ensuring the cuticles are all going in the same direction, which is why Remy hair extensions are of a higher quality!

Non Remy Hair

If the hair extensions you are looking at purchasing does not mention Remy hair, chances are it is not Remy Hair. Non Remy Hair is prone to matting and tangling due to the hair cuticles going in all different directions.

Non Remy hair has simply been cut from a person's hair, and collected straight from the floor. The hair cuticles are all going in different directions, therefore it needs to go through a very strong acid bath to remove the cuticle. This process removes a lot of moisture from the hair, leaving it extremely dry and brittle.

The hair is then coated with silicone conditioners to make it appear soft and shiny. Once the hair has been washed a few times, the silicone coating washes off too, leaving the hair extremely dry and brittle.

IN A NUTSHELL - Non Remy hair has been fundamentally chemically damaged, and is often used in the making of low grade, cheap hair extensions. They are prone to dryness, matting and tangling.

TIP ... ALWAYS purchase Remy Hair Extensions if you want them to last past the first few washes!

HAIR SOURCES

There are many different places/countries human hair is sourced for manufacturing of hair extensions, wigs, and other hair systems. The ones that I discuss, are most widely used for high quality hair extensions. Not all human hair is suitable for manufacturing of hair extensions due to the chemical processes the hair undergoes.

Indian Remy Hair

Indian Remy Hair has its own inherent advantages for use in hair extensions, and is by far the largest source of hair for hair extensions.

It is simultaneously thin and strong and is commonly used in the manufacturing of higher quality hair extensions. The hair comes from Indian widows, who are required to shave their heads, and then put through an osmosis process where the colour pigment is removed. Then over a period of several weeks the colour pigment is saturated back into the hair cuticles with over 54 colour options.

European Remy Hair

European Remy Hair is a popular form of hair used in hair extensions. It has a straight and soft texture. Adequate care must be taken as the market is flooded with fakes. As European Remy Hair is lighter in colour it doesn't go through the same chemical process as Indian Remy Hair which means it is in better condition, and is used in making higher quality human hair. European Remy hair can last a very long time, if cared for properly. There is however due to a worldwide shortage (at the time of writing this book), a lack of European Remy Hair, and it is not currently being used in the producing of hair extensions.

Virgin Remy Hair

Virgin Remy Hair is also known as Virgin Cuticle Hair is the HIGHEST QUALITY hair on the market! It is 100% Natural human hair (uncoloured/unprocessed hair), with all the cuticles intact. NO damage to cuticles, and each cuticle layer is in the same direction, making Virgin Remy Hair Extensions the HIGHEST QUALITY available!

As I mentioned earlier there is a widespread misconception that soft and silky hair is the best quality, so make sure you understand hair type and quality. Real Virgin Remy hair can last a very long time if you care for them properly.

Remember, hair extensions can be made soft and silky through the use of certain conditioners or by coating them in silicone oils during manufacturing (but they will wash out). It is not until after you have washed your hair extensions a couple of times, or until you have used your straightening irons on your hair extensions that you can see the differences in hair quality. This is why purchasing from a reputable supplier is so important.

HAIR GRADING

The "A" Grading system is a standard used by companies to advise manufactures/factories how thick they want the ends of their hair extensions.

The grade of your hair extensions refers not to the quality or type of the hair but to the thickness of the hair extensions to the ends, the higher the grade the thicker they are at the ends.

Companies that advertise Hair Extensions without specifying how full the hair will be at the ends quite often don't understand the product they are selling or supplying to the end user. Be sure to check this when buying Hair Extensions as some companies may supply you less than what you are actually paying for, and your hair extensions may arrive very thin and spindly at the ends.

The grading system below is a common grading system used for hair extensions, however some companies may use a slightly different system.

Double Drawn

Quite simply, Double Drawn is the highest grade available, giving you fullness and body to the ends of your hair extensions. Double Drawn means that the hair collected has been bundled together and has manually had all the shorter hairs in the bundle removed, so that all the hairs are close to the same length. This process is done twice (hence the name Double Drawn) to ensure the extensions will appear much thicker and not wispy or spindly at the ends.

Obviously this process is quite time consuming, and therefore hair extensions that have been through this process are generally more expensive.

Double Drawn hair is also sometimes referred to as Even 7's, or 7A Grade.

The Grading System

Hair extension thickness starts at A Grade, this is the lowest grade available (very spindly at the ends) through to 7A Grade (also known as Double Drawn, this is the highest grade available). Double Drawn hair extensions means 85-90% of the hair is the same length all the way to the ends of your human hair extensions.

As I mentioned earlier some suppliers may use a variation of this grading system, but they will still have a system in place to notify their factory how thick they want the extensions to the ends. So if you are wanting thickness to the ends of your hair extensions, it is important you check this out.

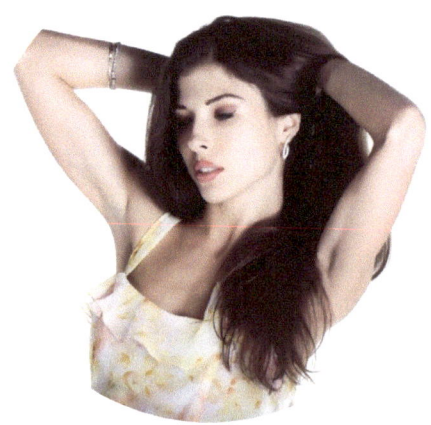

HAIR WEIGHT

When looking at hair weight find out the actual hair weight (net weight). You would be surprised at how much attachments, clips and even packaging can weight ... and you don't want to be mislead.

If you have naturally fine thin hair, then you probably won't want extensions that are too heavy in weight 90-110 grams (depending on length) will most probably be enough. However if you have thick hair you will want a heavy pack 120-140grams(again depending on the length you purchase).

Hair Extensions that are 160+ grams in weight can cause headaches due to the amount of hair weight you are adding to your hair. Therefore optimal weight for hair extensions is 90-140 grams, depending on how thick your own hair is. Also by adding too much hair, you can cause damage to your own natural hair.

As you can see hair extensions are quite complex, understanding:

1. Hair Quality (affects longevity of your extensions)
2. Where the hair is sourced from (affects longevity of your extensions)
3. Hair Grade (volume and thickness at the ends)

Quite simply the old saying if "it seems too good to be true, then it probably is" definitely applies when shopping for hair extensions.

TIP ... Don't just look for high weight extensions, you need to look at the grade also, if you purchase high weight extensions, with a low grade, you will simply end up with the bulk of the hair at the top of the weft, and not much hair at the ends.

Look for a good hair weight, and high grade, so the hair distribution is even over the length of the your hair extensions, to achieve natural fullness.

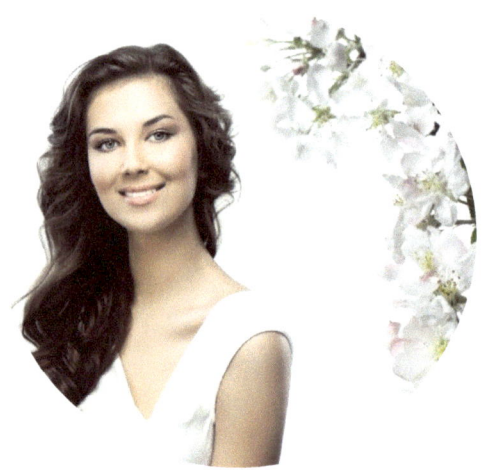

HAIR EXTENSION METHODS

There are many methods of hair extensions from clip in extensions that you simply install yourself at home in minutes through to permanent extensions.

When purchasing hair extensions you need to understand what you are trying to achieve and your lifestyle.

The more common methods used in the industry are:

Clip in Hair Extensions

These are made up from wefts of hair with clips attached. You simply clip them in your hair, and at the end of the day/night remove them again. A full head of clip in extensions usually come in 7-8 piece packs. They are generally non damaging to your hair. They must be removed before sleeping.

They are relatively low maintenance, and require less washing and care than permanent extensions.

Permanent Hair Extensions

All forms of permanent hair extensions require maintenance, as your hair grows your extensions will need to be repositioned back closer to your scalp. Permanent hair extensions when applied correctly should not be visible, and look very natural in your hair.

TIP ... When using permanent hair extensions over long periods of time it is always good to give your hair and scalp a break for a month or two. Invest in clip in extensions for these in between times.

Tape Hair Extensions

This is my personal favourite technique for hair extensions. These are super comfortable, you won't even know you have them in, and they are quick to install (45 minutes - 1 hour).

These are Seamless wefts of hair extensions (normally approx 4cm in width) that come pre-taped. They sit very flat in your head, giving a very natural look.

Tape hair extensions are very light weight and do not put much strain on your natural hair or scalp, as your hair falls in its natural position (the same way it grows) between two tape hair extensions. A section of your natural hair is effectively sandwiched between two tape hair extensions.

I found this to be the most comfortable form of permanent hair extensions.

Tape Hair Extensions are re-usable. They are easily removed with tape hair extension remover (normally a citrus remover), and then re-attached by applying more tape to the top of the extensions, more commonly known as Tape Tabs.

Tape hair extensions will need to be maintained approximately every 6-8 weeks.

Micro Ring/Micro Loop

These are small metal rings, lined with silicone inside, that have a small amount of hair attached to it. Your natural hair is pulled through the metal ring using a loop and then the metal ring clamped with pliers shut.

This method can be uncomfortable to sleep on for the first few nights until you get use to the metal rings.

When it comes time for the hair extensions to be moved or taken out, pliers are used to open the metal rings.

You need to make sure you don't stretch your maintenance visits out too long with this method, otherwise as your hair grows, there is more movement in the scalp area, and you can get hair matting at the scalp, as the micro rings can become tangled.

Micro Ring method needs to be maintained approximately every 6-8 weeks.

Weaving

Your natural hair is braided into corn rows and then a weft of hair extension is sewn into the corn row using a needle and thread.

Weaving is generally better for people with very thick hair, as the strain on the scalp if the corn rows are two tight or if the wefts are too heavy can cause the hair to fall out from the root.

Weaving would have to be the easiest form of permanent hair extensions to remove. You simply cut the thread securing the weft to your natural hair and they're out!

Micro Weaving

This technique combines the traditional weaving technique with micro ring. Whereby wefts of hair are attached to your natural hair and secured by metal micro rings.

This hair extension method is also quite quick to apply taking normally 60-90minutes.

Micro Weave extensions require maintenance approximately every 6 weeks.

Fusion

(Also known as Keratin Tip or Keratin Bonded Extensions)

With this technique, it is very time consuming (hours to install a full head of hair) a machine similar to a hot glue gun is used to attach strands of hair extensions to your natural hair, sometimes in this method the extensions are pre-tipped with a keratin adhesive, and then a heat clamp is used to melt the pre-tip Keratin to attach the extension to your natural hair.

This method requires maintenance approximately every 2months, because of the glue and the heat it is more damaging to your natural hair than other hair extension methods.

 It is extremely important that you seek a professional that is well trained in fusion (bonded) hair extensions.

Hair extension methods involving glue need to be carefully considered, due to the risk of damage to your scalp and natural hair if they are not done correctly, or if your hair is weak.

IN SUMMARY

I believe it is extremely important to love and nurture your hair. How your hair looks and reacts will largely depend on how you treat it. The same goes with your hair extensions, both need TLC.

Hair extensions can dramatically improve your hair and overall image by adding volume, length and highlights.

When shopping for hair extensions:

1. choose a hair extension method that is right for you
2. choose a quality hair extension supplier, a company that you feel has extensive knowledge of hair extensions (quality, sourcing, grading etc)

Remember your hair is not a living organ, it can't repair itself, so love it and look after it! Your hair is your crown and glory.

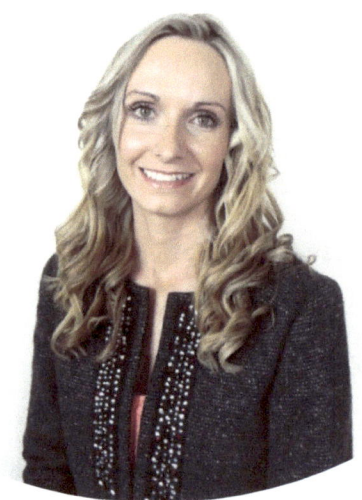

Mandy Allen, Director Hollywood Glamour Hair Extensions

A NOTE OF THANKS

They say behind every successful woman, is a great man! I would also like to add, a great family!

Thank you to my partner Gavin, and to my family for always encouraging me to pursue my dreams and passion.

By T.P Just

~~~

Copyright © 2010 by Terence Just. All rights reserved.

Get All The Books In The Series:

Animal Peculiarity Volume 1 Part [1-8]
Animal Peculiarity Volume 2 Part [1-8]
Animal Peculiarity Volume 3 Part [1-8]
<u>Just Enterprises</u>

Table of Contents